How to Strengthen Your Immune System

Discover the Best Immunity Boosting Foods, Vitamins, Herbs, and Other Effective Ways to Strengthen the Immune System

by Louise Berlitz

Table of Contents

Introduction 1

Chapter 1: Getting Rid of Toxins 7

Chapter 2: How to Structure Your Diet 13

Chapter 3: Maintaining a Healthy Lifestyle 27

Chapter 4: How to Deal with Stress 33

Chapter 5: Improving Your Physique 37

Chapter 6: How to Keep Your Home Clean 45

Conclusion 51

Introduction

To some extent, your health and quality of life are determined by genetics and the environment in which you live. However, to an even greater extent, your overall health, quality of life, and longevity are largely determined by the choices you make each day, which are entirely under your control.

If you haven't already started taking responsibility for your actions and their effects, it may be time to do so. A healthy lifestyle can help prevent a variety of diseases — such as heart disease, cancer, and diabetes – all of which are significant causes of premature deaths. Strengthening your health and boosting your immune system also requires that you make some small and gradual but important changes in your life and in your diet. This doesn't have to be an abrupt change where you stop enjoying what you like to eat altogether. A healthy diet simply means eating a wide variety of naturally occurring foods and maintaining your weight at a desirable level.

To boost your immune system, you will also need to engage in sports or some form of exercise or physical activity that will strengthen your body. Regular moderate exercise – as simple as just taking a walk – can lead to a gradual but significant improvement in your physical condition as well as improved mental energy and alertness.

This book is designed to provide you important yet easy to follow guidelines for healthy living. For instance, you will find information on how to start a healthy diet based on a wide variety of fresh fruits, whole grains, and fresh vegetables. You will also find tips on how to start a suitable fitness program that is fun and sustainable. These steps and tips may sound simple and they most certainly are, but therein lies the beauty of it: By keeping things simple, this will ultimately lead you to positive improvements in your immune system and your overall health that can be implemented immediately yet will remain effective throughout the long term. Let's get started!

© Copyright 2015 by Miafn LLC - All rights reserved.

This document is geared towards providing reliable information in regards to the topic and issue covered. The publication is sold with the idea that the publisher is not required to render accounting, officially permitted, or otherwise, qualified services. If advice is necessary, legal or professional, a practiced individual in the profession should be ordered.

- From a Declaration of Principles which was accepted and approved equally by a Committee of the American Bar Association and a Committee of Publishers and Associations.

In no way is it legal to reproduce, duplicate, or transmit any part of this document in either electronic means or in printed format. Recording of this publication is strictly prohibited and any storage of this document is not allowed unless with written permission from the publisher. All rights reserved.

The information provided herein is stated to be truthful and consistent, in that any liability, in terms of inattention or otherwise, by any usage or abuse of any policies, processes, or directions contained within is solely and completely the responsibility of the recipient reader. Under no circumstances will any legal responsibility or blame be held against the publisher for any reparation, damages, or monetary loss due to the information herein, either directly or indirectly.

Respective authors own all copyrights not held by the publisher.

The information herein is offered for informational purposes solely, and is universal as so. The presentation of the information is without contract or any type of guarantee assurance.

The trademarks that are used are without any consent, and the publication of the trademark is without permission or backing by the trademark owner. All trademarks and brands within this book are for clarifying purposes only and are the owned by the owners themselves, not affiliated with this document.

Chapter 1: Getting Rid of Toxins

Do you often feel bloated? Do you sweat profusely? Are you suffering from debilitating headaches? Do you often have difficulty concentrating? Do you keep forgetting simple day-to-day things? Do you have frequent mood swings? Do you constantly suffer from allergic reactions? Do you have very poor digestion?

These are classic signs of toxic overload. If you experience any of these symptoms, coupled with feeling constant tiredness and a marked intolerance to fat, then you may be suffering from toxic overload. However, it is possible to get rid of those toxins and feel healthier by detoxifying and cleansing your whole body in a few simple steps and within just a few days.

Detoxifying and cleansing your body of toxins will lead to better health, a better immune system and a more energetic and revitalized you. Some of the benefits of detoxification are a well-toned body, loss of several pounds of weight, better digestion and a big boost to your immune system. Detoxification allows you to clear out all the toxins and poisons that have accumulated inside your body over the years.

But before you embark on a detoxification program, you are strongly advised to consult with your medical practitioner. If you are pregnant or breastfeeding, or undergoing medical treatment for a serious ailment, for instance, it is best that you do not embark on a detoxification program. Some examples of these ailments are diabetes, heart conditions, anemia, cancer and other serious and life-threatening medical disorders. If you are underweight or under a lot of stress, you are advised not to start a detox program. It is always recommended that you check with your doctor or nurse before going on any form of detoxification program.

Once you get the approval from your doctor, adopt a positive attitude from the start of the detox program. In order to succeed in the program, you must always keep focused on why you are doing it, whether you want a well-toned body or to feel fit and healthy or to improve your blood circulation.

At the start of each day of the detox program, practice breathing deeply and correctly as this is a very important element of your detox program. It helps to cleanse, relax and energize your body. Start by lying down on the floor of a quiet room and place both hands on your abdomen. Then slowly begin to breathe in through your nose and count to five and feel your belly expanding under your fingertips. Hold your breath for a few seconds and exhale up to a count of ten. Repeat this cycle several times until you feel a calm spread over you, and you begin to feel more relaxed. Continue each day of the detox program with a good frame of mind to keep yourself motivated and excited about the positive effects of cleansing and detoxifying your body and mind.

One of the basics of detoxifying your body is to eat at least three well-chosen meals. You must also allow at least a five–hour window between meals to allow your body enough time to process your food before the next meal. Fresh fruits and vegetables are a major part of detoxifying your body. The abundance of vitamins and minerals contained in fruits and vegetables are a major factor in boosting your immune system while you flush out the toxins from your system.

Detoxing, however, is not a diet program. Rather, think of it as spring cleaning your body and ridding it of all the toxins accumulated in your organs due to years of poor eating habits. To do this, your body needs at least ten to twelve glasses of water daily. Avoid drinking coffee, alcoholic drinks, carbonated or fizzy beverages. Drinking that much water every day may seem a lot at first, but your body will soon adjust. If drinking plain water sounds boring and does not give you the incentive to drink, try adding lemon, lime, honey, and ginger for flavor and for added health benefits. You may also opt to drink herbal or organic teas like green tea. Just remember to always consume plenty of clean and healthy fluids

Plan your meals every day while remembering to adhere to the five-hour window of fasting between meals. Always consume at least three portions of fruits, four portions of vegetables, two portions of fish, four portions of nuts, four portions of salads and one portion of grains like brown rice. Try to eat the last meal of the day not later than seven in the evening to allow your body to digest your meal fully before you go to bed. Before you go to bed, do some deep breathing again until you feel calm and relaxed and ready for a good night's sleep.

Detoxifying yourself also allows the dirty air you breathe in to be cleansed from your system. By eliminating those toxins, you allow your body to return to over-all good health thereby improving your immune system, your blood circulation, as well as your body's ability to heal and repair itself. Flushing out the toxins—from the fatty and high-sodium foods you consumed to the pollutants in the environment—ensures that your body gets a maintenance check much like a car's regular check-up to keep it working efficiently.

Chapter 2: How to Structure Your Diet

Now that you are more aware of the basics of detoxifying your body, it's time to get serious about changing your existing habits to see a marked improvement in your health. A healthy diet does more than match your energy intake to energy output. It provides all the elements required for the optimal performance of your immune system. Thus, one crucial step is to eat and drink sensibly. Learn to consume a great variety of healthy foods like organic fruits and vegetables. You may at first think that opting for healthier food choices will limit your options, but you will actually be spoiled for choice.

There is no lack of healthy and organic food choices in restaurants and the grocery store these days because of the growing awareness about eating healthy and going green. If you eat a balanced diet from a wide selection of naturally occurring foods as opposed to packaged processed foods you are on your way to a positive lifestyle change that will improve your quality of life.

Eating a balanced, adequate diet helps promote good health in many ways. More and more people are not only eating nutritionally balanced diets but are taking the green and organic path to healthy eating. Going green and eating organic foods allows you to trounce old and bad eating habits based on a diet—filled with grease, more meat than you need and all those empty calories from highly processed foods—that makes you overfed and yet grossly undernourished.

Today, many people fit that profile. This kind of malnutrition stems from consuming the wrong kinds of foods. On average, adults and children alike generally eat only one serving of fruit or vegetable daily, if they consume any fruit or vegetable at all. The stresses and demands of daily life also lead many to limit themselves to very poor food choices that usually come in a box, a plastic bag or a frozen container.

Probably the biggest problem with the average person's diet these days is that too much food is consumed with far more calories than are actually needed by the body. Worse yet, the average person does not even burn half of the calories consumed because of a very sedentary lifestyle. The result is a generally overweight, even obese, population. Maintaining an adequate level of physical activity is essential to maintaining your weight. Ready to eat convenience foods usually have very little or no nutritional value and yet they pack a lot of empty calories, unhealthy fats, oils and sugars.

Now that you have embarked on a detoxification program, it is also time to recalibrate your eating program to a healthier one, one filled with healthier and greener options. When you start feeding yourself a nutritious diet, you are now giving your body the building blocks to a healthier and better you.

Eating better and healthier gives you more energy, greater physical well-being, improved mood, strengthened immunity, increased brain power and enhanced concentration, fewer everyday illnesses, reduced risk of serious diseases like cancer, reduced risk of obesity and its corresponding ailments. Choose healthier options like brown rice and beans instead of fast food, deep-fried chicken or some other nutritionally vacant foods. Make every bite count from now on.

A healthy diet contains adequate quantities of six groups of essential substances such as proteins, carbohydrates and fats, all of which contain calories, that is, they produce nutrients that produce energy. You also need fiber, vitamins and minerals for a healthy diet. Although fiber, vitamins and minerals are essential to a healthy diet and to good health, they do not contain any calories.

In addition, you need plenty of water, without which life is impossible. A human being deprived of both food and drink usually can survive for only 4 or 5 days, but can live for as long as two months on liquids alone. Your body is made up of about 65% to 80% water. You lose about two liters every day in the moisture of the breath you exhale, sweat, urine and stool. Lost fluid must be replenished. As mentioned in the last chapter, even if you find it difficult at first to drink ten glasses of water daily, it is important to increase your fluid intake, and to maintain this daily intake to help flush out any impurities.

To improve your overall health as well as to lower your risk of developing cancer, high blood pressure and diabetes, you must eat a variety of foods and maintain a healthy weight. Choose a diet low in total fat, saturated fat and cholesterol. Choose a diet with plenty of vegetables, fruits and grain products. Use sugar only in moderation and choose the less refined ones such as brown or muscovado or coconut sugar. Avoid salt if you can. If you have to, use salt or sodium only in moderation. Make sure that fresh fruits, whole grains and vegetables are a major part of your diet.

Monitor your protein intake and make sure you eat lean white meat instead of red meat and fatty portions or cuts. Proteins are the chemical compounds that form the basis of living matter. You need a regular daily intake of protein for the repair, replacement, growth and full function of your body. Peas, beans and other legumes, as well as grains, meat, fish, eggs and cheese provide proteins, but beware since meats and cheeses can be high in fat. Also bear in mind that if you eat more protein than your body needs, the extra protein is converted into glucose and provides energy or is converted to fat and stored by your body.

Fats are found in plant foods such as olives and peanuts as well as in animal products. Fats provide energy and minute quantities of fat are also used for repair and growth of your body. In addition, fats make food palatable and filling. Depending on chemical composition, fats are either saturated or unsaturated; a distinction that matters primarily because eating saturated fats is thought to increase the amount of cholesterol in the blood and cause serious health problems for your body.

Animal fats, especially those in milk, butter, cheese and meat are mostly saturated and may be partly responsible for the development of atherosclerosis. The fat in fish and some vegetable oils is largely unsaturated. In chicken and turkey, most of the fat is in the skin. From the standpoint of health, the better fats are polyunsaturated and monounsaturated, provided by avocado, olive oil, and other vegetable oils. In cooking, it is advisable to substitute these liquid oils for solid fats (saturated and trans fats).

Avoid canned and processed foods as much as possible because they contain many additives and preservatives. Consume fish instead of meat. Fish is a perfect food because it contains all the vital proteins your body needs. Fish is healthier when prepared fresh from the source rather than frozen because freezing depletes fish of essential nutrients. Refrain from eating fish in brine as well because of the excess salt. If you have to choose from canned fish, choose those preserved in vegetable oil.

A healthy diet must have the right amount of carbohydrates, which are chemicals that contain carbon, hydrogen and oxygen. All the foods that we think of as being either starchy or sugary contain a high proportion of carbohydrates. Some examples are sugar, bread, pasta, rice, potatoes and cereals. These foods are our main source of energy and some of them contribute other essential elements of a balanced diet, such as vitamins and minerals. For example, potatoes and whole grain bread contain fiber, cereals contain protein and whole grain bread is also a good source of iron.

Fiber is also a very important part of a healthy diet. The human digestive tract is unable to digest fiber, which is plant material such as cellulose and pectin that is found in unrefined cereals, fruit, vegetables and legumes. Fiber is very important because it provides bulk to help the large intestine efficiently carry away body wastes. Fiber may also help prevent cancer of the large intestine and diverticular disease.

If you have a juicer, you can make your own fresh juice using any fresh fruits you fancy. Some homemade fruit juices you can try are apple, grape, grapefruit, lemon, lime, mango, melon, papaya, peach, pear, pineapple, strawberry and watermelon. You may also try home-made vegetable juices, or combine them with fruit juices to add variety. Some vegetables you should try are beet, carrot, celery, cucumber and watercress.

These homemade fruit and vegetable juices make delicious drinks that pack a lot of vitamins and minerals. The vitamins contained in foods are essentially chemicals. Your body can make small amounts of some vitamins, such as vitamin D, which is made in the skin when exposed to sunlight, but most vitamins can be obtained only from food or supplements.

Anyone who eats a varied diet of fresh fruits and vegetables, grains, dairy products, fish and meat generally gets enough vitamins. However, some findings suggest that the average American diet does not contain enough vitamin A and C year-round or enough vitamin D in the winter months. The best solution is not for you to take supplements, but instead, you should change your diet so that you eat fresh, vitamin-rich foods.

If you eat additional fresh fruits and vegetables, your new routine will provide enough vitamins A, C, D, and E to avoid osteoporosis and possibly cancer. Also, fruits and vegetables contain valuable fiber and reduce your appetite for less-healthy fats and sugars.

By changing your eating habits and eating healthy foods regularly now that you are on your detoxification program, your energy levels will be maintained throughout the day. Now you will feel more alert, healthy and energized.

The Food Pyramid is a simple and general plan for eating sensibly every day. You can use the pyramid to choose the right amounts of all the foods that are essential to a well-balanced diet. Following these recommendations will help ensure that you get enough protein, carbohydrates, vitamins, minerals and fiber every day while also limiting your intake of fats, cholesterol, sugar and salt or sodium. Note that one serving is not the same as one helping, which usually contains more than one serving.

Your body also needs at least 20 minerals in your diet. But only iron, calcium, iodine and sodium are of major nutritional importance. An apparently reasonable diet may not be deficient in iron, calcium or iodine. Foods such as bread, however, may be fortified with added iron and calcium. In parts of the world where the soil is deficient in iodine, it is often added to salt. A well-balanced diet usually provides enough iron, calcium and iodine.

You should limit your daily intake of fats, oils and sweets. Foods from this group include butter, margarine, vegetable oils, salad dressings, soft drinks and candy. These foods are generally high in calories and low in nutritional value. Fats should account for no more than 30% of your total daily intake of calories. Note that sugars and fats can in fact be present in all of the other food groups.

You may have 2 to 3 servings per day of meat, poultry, fish, dry beans, eggs or nuts. This means you can eat 2 to 3 ounces of meat, fish or poultry every day. You may also consume a third of one serving of 1 egg, 2 tablespoons of peanut butter and 1/2 cup of cooked dry beans daily. Foods from this food group provide protein, vitamin B and minerals such as iron. Go easy on the nuts because they are high in fat. Choose lean cuts of red meat and trim all visible fat. Remove skin from poultry. Limit yourself to three or four eggs per week to cut down on cholesterol.

You may consume 6 to 11 servings of bread, cereal, rice or pasta. Foods from this group provide carbohydrates, vitamins, minerals and fiber. Choose whole grain products. Read package labels to check for added amounts of fat, sugar and sodium, especially in ready to eat cereals. Watch out for added fats, cholesterol and sugar in spreads, salad dressings and toppings.

You can eat around 2 to 3 servings of dairy such as a cup of milk, yogurt, natural or processed cheese. Foods from this group provide calcium, protein, vitamins and minerals. Choose skim, low-fat, or non-fat milk and dairy products.

To maintain your daily dose of natural vitamins and minerals, you also need to eat 3 to 5 servings of vegetables per day. Foods from this group are low in fat and provide vitamins such as vitamins A and C, minerals such as iron and fiber. Choose plenty of dark green, leafy vegetables, deep yellow vegetables and legumes such as peas and beans. When preparing vegetable dishes, use low fat or nonfat dressings and topping to limit added fats and cholesterol.

You also need to eat 2 to 4 servings per day of fruit. Foods from this food group are low in fat and sodium and provide vitamins such as A and C, minerals such as potassium and fiber. Choose fresh whole fruits whenever possible. If canned fruit, then choose only fruit packed in its own juice. Read package labels to check for added sugar in canned fruits and canned or bottled juices.

Many people eat too much sodium or salt. Salt is known to increase the risk of heart disease for people who already have high blood pressure. Many people add salt to food in cooking and at the table out of habit. Taste your food before salting it and you will discover that your food tastes better without added salt.

To maintain a healthy weight, try to eat the lowest number of servings recommended for each food group.

Some special considerations will, however, require some changes in daily food requirements. For instance, teenagers, young adults and women who are pregnant or breastfeeding need at least 3 servings of milk and other dairy products each day. Sedentary women and older people only need to consume about 1,600 calories per day while children, teenage girls, active women and sedentary men need to take in about 2,200 calories per day. Teenage boys, active men and very active women need to take in about 2,800 calories per day. If you are not sure about how many calories you need per day, talk to your physician.

There are also special diets that can reduce the risk of serious illnesses such as cancer. Research shows that you can choose a diet that is nutritious and that will help lower your risk of getting cancer. We have been emphasizing the importance of reducing the amount of fat you eat. Make an effort to reduce your fat intake to no more than 30% of your total calories. A varied diet that is low in fat and cholesterol but high in fiber can significantly lower the risk of cancer. Choose fresh fruit and vegetables that are in season. Eat more fruits, vegetables and whole grain products for all the benefits previously mentioned.

Growing your own organic garden can also help you eat better and boost your immunity from diseases. Organic vegetables are grown naturally without using any chemicals or employing any procedure which kills bacteria or acts as a preservative. Thus, planting a garden at home or in your community will ensure safer foods and food security. If you buy natural produce, carefully choose the food you buy. Some organic foods are worth the extra money you pay for them because they have been proven to be safer, tastier and more nutritious than conventionally grown kinds. Buy organic whenever possible. Organic food means it is 95% organic. Food labeled all-natural does not mean it is organic.

When detoxing and changing your eating habits, it is also important for you to change your cooking methods. In fact the less cooking done in food preparation the better it is to preserve the nutrients and vitamins. If you still prefer your vegetables slightly cooked, avoid boiling, slow cooking or frying them. Instead, use other methods such as broiling, stir frying or just popping them into the microwave. This way, the vegetables retain their nutrients and are far tastier.

Chapter 3: Maintaining a Healthy Lifestyle

Your good health and longevity can be attributed to several factors such as lifestyle, environment and genetics. Living a healthy lifestyle is one of the most important things you can control to prevent illness. After you have successfully detoxed your whole system, you should immediately feel the positive effects in your body and the way you feel.

Start and end each day with the deep breathing exercises described in chapter 1. Practice breathing deeply and correctly to continually cleanse your body of toxins and to help you to relax

Start your healthy and consistent daily regimen by quitting any bad habits that you have. If you smoke, quit immediately. Smoking causes not only lung cancer but also heart disease and other forms of cancer such as mouth, esophagus, throat, bladder and cervix. Smoking also accelerates aging of your skin, your bones and your lungs.

If you drink alcohol, minimize or totally eliminate your intake of alcoholic beverages. If you cannot totally avoid drinking, drink only in moderation. Do not drink if you are undergoing medical treatment or if you are stressed or pregnant. Do not drink if you are driving or operating heavy equipment or machinery. If you have a problem controlling your drinking, ask for help from your doctor. You may also ask for help from support groups like Alcoholics Anonymous. The same is applicable if you have a problem with substance abuse. You should ask for help or get yourself into a reliable drug rehabilitation facility.

See your doctor regularly for medical check-ups and screening. Screening allows you to detect any disease while it is in the early and treatable stage. Always consult your doctor about any symptoms or medical complaints.

Maintain good dental health as well. A professional cleaning done every six months will help protect gums as well as teeth from the ravages of plaque. Fluoride treatments will also strengthen tooth enamel. You may also ask your dentist to apply protective sealant to chewing surfaces, which will fill the pits and crevices in the chewing surfaces and prevent the trapping of debris and the colonization of decay-causing bacteria. Get into the habit of brushing three times a day, especially within 20 minutes after meals. Replace your toothbrush after two months or after a bout of illness. Rinse your toothbrush thoroughly after each use and keep it in a holder rather than lying around where it can pick up bacteria. Good dental health that lasts a lifetime depends on good daily dental care.

Keep your body fit and trim by exercising regularly. Choose a fitness regimen that suits your lifestyle and schedule. Do your preferred exercise or sport for at least one hour per day and at least five days a week. Get a fitness buddy if you have difficulty getting motivated and staying on track every day.

People who exercise are stronger and have greater endurance than people who do not. A wonderful benefit of exercise includes protection from coronary heart disease. Regular, moderate exercise will make your heart and lungs stronger and more resilient. Although exercise may not decrease the amount of fat deposits in the arteries, it may increase the good cholesterol, widen the arteries and make the complete blockage, such as that from a clot, less likely.

Joints that are exercised regularly stay flexible and healthy. Brisk walking and swimming are good exercises to help keep your joints moving smoothly. Exercise builds the strength of bones by stimulating bone-building cells to create new bone.

Exercise improves your bone strength no matter what your age. This is especially important for women who are of menopausal age when a lack of estrogen may lead to osteoporosis. Exercise will help build up the bones to help protect against fractures in the future. Exercise makes people feel good. People who exercise regularly feel healthy and are less likely to become depressed.

Maintain a healthy weight range based on your age and height, to minimize your risk for heart disease and other serious diseases. If you are overweight now, try harder to lose the excess weight with proper diet and discipline. Once you have gotten the hang of it, try hard to maintain your new lifestyle, and you will soon see the positive results that will boost your immunity and positively impact your quality of life.

Chapter 4: How to Deal with Stress

Any significant change in your daily routine, will have some impact on your system, and whether good or bad, it can be stressful. However, an occasional period of stress is usually distinct from other emotional problems which may have to be treated professionally.

A death in the family or loss of a close friend, divorce, financial difficulties, serious illness and incessant worry are all part and parcel of life. But as everyday stresses accumulate, you may become increasingly susceptible to serious physical illness, behavioral disturbances and grave emotional problems. When several stressful events occur at the same time, the normal stressful things become serious stressors and you may suffer from severe stress, sometimes even leading to serious physical injuries as result of an accident.

There is no way that anyone can avoid stress altogether. The key is how to cope with stress and manage those stressors in your life so that stress does not eventually cause serious and debilitating illnesses such as cancer and heart disease.

In order to cope successfully with tensions and difficulties in life, you first need to have a healthy attitude as well as a healthy body, and manage your stress constructively in order to protect your mental and physical wellbeing. The best you can do is to minimize the negative impact of stress in your life by focusing on the present and not dwelling on the past. Think about how you can make concrete steps to ensure that the future will be manageable instead of just worrying about what will happen. Deal with your problems one at a time and look for the best solutions for each problem individually. Do not complain and worry about your difficulties, but endeavor to act on the best possible solution you can find. Make it a point to take deep breaths to calm and relax your troubled mind. If you need professional help, get help immediately. The best way to cope with stress is to deal with it positively.

Chapter 5: Improving Your Physique

In the last four chapters, you were reminded of the importance of exercise in managing your stress and improving your health. You have been encouraged to change your lifestyle, to eat right and find ways to cope with stressful events in your life. Exercise is the ideal way to get your body system going and to further increase your metabolic rate. Note however, that certain exercises and fitness programs will be better suited to you than others. Before you decide on a fitness regimen, focus for a while on how your body works and how important each organ is to improving your immune system and your overall health.

Your Brain—Begin with the health and good functioning of your brain. Studies show that the best thing you can do for your brain is to get enough sleep. If you get less than the amount of sleep your body needs to rest and regenerate, you compromise your ability to perform well mentally and you compromise your brain's ability to function and store memories. To boost your brain function and generate new cells in the memory area, you need a minimum amount of 15 minutes of aerobic exercise three times a week. You also need to be smart about the kinds of foods you eat for better brain function. Omega-3 fatty acids help keep the brain healthy and may even ward off age-related damage. At least five servings a week of omega-3 rich foods such as salmon, sardines, walnuts and grass-fed beef are recommended in order to keep your brain healthy and functioning at optimum levels.

Your Heart—Your heart is the main muscle that you need to keep in top shape. Heart disease is the leading cause of deaths in both men and women in most countries. If too much good food has been your indulgence, then the first order of the day is to reduce your girth, or waistline. Research directly links belly fat to hardening of the arteries which can lead to heart disease. Thin your middle by avoiding processed foods because the trans fats they contain create more belly fat than other forms of dietary fat. Get your blood pressure and cholesterol levels checked at least annually, especially if you have a family history of heart disease and your numbers are high. Your blood pressure should not be higher than 120/80 and your total cholesterol should be under 200. If left unchecked, high cholesterol and high blood pressure can clog your arteries and increase your risk of a heart attack.

Your Liver—Your liver is a multitasking organ that performs more than 5,000 functions including storing vitamins and minerals and straining alcohol and other toxins out of your system. Drinking alcoholic beverages injures your liver's cells and increases your risk of liver disease such as cirrhosis, cancer and liver failure. But the largest contributing factor to liver disease is obesity. Fatty deposits in your liver can cause inflammation and scarring which can contribute to cirrhosis and cancer. To help reduce this risk, incorporate weight training in your fitness regimen and include protein in every meal to help add lean muscle to your frame. Lastly, do not engage in unprotected sex because Hepatitis B and C can be transmitted through unprotected sex.

Your Lungs—Your lungs don't just help you breathe by taking in oxygen into your body. They also trap viruses, bacteria and other airborne particles. So the healthier your lungs are, the less likely you are to get sick. To keep your lungs healthy, quit smoking if you smoke. At the risk of sounding repetitive, I will reiterate, that smoking is the leading cause of lung cancer. Lung cancer kills more people than breast, prostate and colon cancer combined. Studies also show that being overweight is bad for your lungs. When you're heavy, the excess fat on your chest wall forces your respiratory system to have to work harder. Losing 10% of your excess body weight, if you are overweight by 40 pounds or more, improves lung capacity by 5%.

Your Pancreas—Sandwiched between your stomach and your spleen, this organ creates insulin, the hormone that regulates your blood sugar and makes you feel either sated and energized or ravenous and shaky, depending on how much is in your system. Studies show that people who eat two or more servings of high fiber whole grains a day which is equal to about a cup of high-fiber cereal have a 40% lower risk of developing pancreatic cancer than those who eat one serving or less daily. So load up on fiber to keep your pancreas healthy and to reduce the risk of gallstones. Gallstones are tiny pieces of crystallized cholesterol that can cause pancreatitis, a nasty condition that can lead to pancreatic cancer. The steps you take to take care of your other organs such as not smoking, keeping a healthy weight and exercising regularly will keep your pancreas healthy too.

Now that you have taken some steps to take care of your vital organs, you need to focus your attention on choosing a good exercise program for yourself. The best exercise for you is one that you will enjoy and will do regularly. You can start a daily walking routine. Gentle and easy walking stimulates the lungs, the heart, the muscles and even the mind. You may begin your walking routine with ten to fifteen minutes every day for the first two weeks while gradually building up to thirty minutes when you hit the first month of your walking routine. Then you may move up to brisk walking on the second month. You should walk fast enough that you break a slight sweat.

However, you should still continue to consult with your medical practitioner about the best physical form of exercise you need and which would not strain your body too much, particularly if you have been inactive for very long and are just about to start your fitness regimen. If you haven't exercised in a while or are just starting to get physically fit, do not exercise strenuously. Begin gently and ease slowly into your chosen physical routine. If you overdo it, you may overtire your muscles and strain your body. Instead of strengthening your immune system, overexerting yourself may actually create more waste products in your body and strain your lymphatic system.

Choose types of exercise that you enjoy and that you can fit into your schedule. Make it a point to set aside some time to enjoy an invigorating bike ride or some swimming whenever your schedule permits it. If you don't know how to swim or ride a bike, now is a good time to start learning these useful skills. Swimming works most of the major muscle groups and is an excellent aerobic exercise. At the same time, it is very soothing and relaxing to the spine. It is highly recommended for anyone who has a predominantly sedentary type of work and a tendency to suffer from shoulder and back ache.

Whatever exercise you decide to do, you need to start slowly and then build up gradually. Try to find a form of exercise that challenges you physically and also relaxes your mind. Engage in exercise or sport that you will enjoy. Do not choose something you don't like. Exercise should not only be good for you but it should also be fun and enjoyable. Exercise throughout the day for a total of 30 minutes at least 5 times a day every week. Exercise moderately. If you get dizzy or nauseated, or if you feel pain, these may be signs you are straining yourself and overdoing it. Always do warm up stretching exercises before the main exercise session and cool down stretching exercises at the end.

If you prefer cycling or swimming, then go ahead. These are some of the best types of exercise for building muscle endurance and for toning your leg muscles. You may also choose to use a stationary bike in the gym or at your own home. You may also bounce on a trampoline for around five to fifteen minutes daily to help drain your lymphatic system.

Even vigorous housework is a good form of exercise so you can even choose to integrate vigorous housework, like scrubbing floors or washing your car, as part of your daily fitness regimen. Energetic gardening or do-it-yourself work around the house can be good ways to exercise. Many people find that cycling or brisk walking to and from work, or walking up the stairs instead of taking the elevator fits nicely into their everyday routines. The goal is to develop a habit of integrating physical activity into your life so that you look forward to your chosen activity.

Chapter 6: How to Keep Your Home Clean

Achieving a healthy life balance is the key to maintaining your health and boosting your immune system. You not only need to keep your body strong and your mind active, alert and relaxed—you also need to keep everything in your life manageable. To do this, you need to devote quality time to each aspect of your life. You need to occupy yourself and your mind as much as possible in a positive way. When confronted with a difficult life experience, you need to think about your future in terms that you can manage instead of worrying about an unknown future that you have no means of controlling.

If you can't decide where to start in getting your much needed life balance in order to boost your immune system and improve your health, start with the basics like your immediate surroundings. We usually think of our homes as the safest place that we can be but scientific research shows that most walls even in our homes are covered with pathogenic bacteria.

If, like most households, you don't regularly wash and clean your walls and your entire home, you and your family are in danger of health risks from a variety of bacteria and germs. Pathogenic bacteria are a major cause of human death and disease. These bacteria cause infections such as respiratory infections and food-borne illness. Mold in the home is scientifically linked to chronic asthma symptoms as well as chronic coughing, wheezing and other respiratory tract symptoms in otherwise healthy people.

But keeping your home safe and clean is a very tall order. Indeed keeping house is a 25hour/8day job. When you finally find time to clean some portions of the house, you've got another one that needs immediate attention. The amount of clutter in a household, dirty laundry and scattered stuff can be overwhelming.

There is no way of getting around it, unfortunately, but to face the mess and the clutter head on. So start with the bedrooms. The bedroom is the most important part of your home as you spend a third of your life in this room. It is where you sleep, rest, hang out, relax, play and watch TV so naturally things can get messy.

Clean your bedrooms daily or at least weekly. Make up beds every morning. Rotate your mattress to even out the wear on the material. You can also flip the mattress but check the label first. Remove linen then vacuum both sides of the mattress to get rid of dust mites. Air your mattress at least once a month or take it out to your veranda or terrace for sunning. Sunlight also acts as a natural disinfectant. As much as possible avoid using water because moisture may lead to mildew formation. Spot clean using a mild detergent. Wash your pillows at least every other month. Check the label if it is machine washable.

Keep your closet clean to make sure that your clothes remain clean and last longer. Vacuum your closet to remove stray hair, lint and insect larvae. Vacuum all surfaces, corners and the floor.

In the kitchen, maintain optimum cleanliness to minimize the growth of bacteria and avoid the presence of vermin, cockroaches or ants. Clean your fridge inside and out with soft cloth and lukewarm soapy water. Clean up food spills immediately to prevent leaks, uneven cooling and the spread of bacteria. Perform regular cleaning every week to prevent food contamination.

Your bathroom is also one area that needs to be cleaned daily for obvious reasons. All the surfaces must be scrubbed clean with effective cleaning agents to prevent diseases and infection in your home. Clean toilet bowl and seat covers every day. Follow instructions for toilet bowl cleaner and pour necessary amount into the bowl. Focus under the rim as this harbors a lot of germs. Spray disinfectant on toilet seat and toilet seat cover. Regularly mop floors to prevent stains and mildew.

The same goes for the other areas and appliances such as air conditioners in your home. Regularly vacuum or sweep all visible dirt. Vacuum or wash your drapes at least once a week or have them cleaned out thoroughly by professional cleaners at least once a year. If your schedule allows it, take down your curtains every three weeks and throw them in the washing machine or take them to the dry cleaners. Rugs and carpets in your home are dust and dirt magnets so they need regular care and maintenance. Clean your carpet at least every other month.

Keeping all the rooms and areas in your home clean is one way to prevent illness and guarantee that you and your family benefit from the healthy changes you have started to implement.

Conclusion

In this day and age of sound bites and buzz words about staying healthy and keeping fit as well as the advances in science, medicine and technology, people still get sick. In the past, being healthy and having a strong immune system meant working very hard at it, like working up a sweat with extreme sports and workouts or going on a full-on vegetarian diet. These days, the focus has shifted from pumping iron, taking steroids and supplements, and working out to exhaustion, to living a moderate lifestyle with sustainable physical fitness regime.

But every day, our own personal beliefs about health and staying healthy are also shifting from the traditional to what is actually true for each of us. There may be changing beliefs and paradigms in science and technology about how to deal with disease and manage health, but at the end of the day, it all boils down to how you address your personal health issues and being smart about it.

Adjust your eating habits to any changes in your lifestyle or schedule. Decide what unhealthy foods you can live without and then leave them out of your diet. But if they are the things that you really crave, then you don't have to give them up totally. Just eat them in limited quantities.

Healthy eating is not just about following a very strict diet but rather knowing what right foods to eat and how to do portion control to maintain your caloric intake and your weight. The same is true for exercise and sports

Coping with the daily demands of your career and family life are already demanding as it is. Therefore, the key to keeping yourself healthy, maintaining a healthy weight and lifestyle, and boosting your immune system, is to maintain a healthy balance in all aspects of your life.

You need to manage your stress. Keep fit and physically active. Eat healthy and eat only what you need. While you strive to maintain a healthy lifestyle, the demands of your everyday life can often make it difficult for you to sustain these lifestyle changes and habits. Everyday stresses often put your body out of its natural balance and rhythm.

If you are a first time runner, ease yourself into it and train gradually before you decide to join your first marathon. For first-timers, walk for ten minutes then run for one minute. Walk another five minutes and run for one minute. Do that for a week. Then the next week, increase your run time to two minutes and see how it goes for the next two months. If you still do not get the hang of it and decide you don't like it, then try your hand at something else. Maybe you should try swimming or dance classes at the gym.

Read books to help you achieve your goals, or get a coach, or do both. It helps that, in your new path to changing your lifestyle and physical fitness regimen, you choose well and do things properly. If you can, always seek help so you can achieve your personal fitness and health goals while understanding how to do things right and keeping yourself safe and free from injuries.

Determine your personal goals, whether it is beating your illness and boosting your immune system in general or getting to your ideal weight or body mass index. Then, focus on how you will achieve your goals. Do something you really enjoy. If working out at the gym bores you, then take your fitness regimen outdoors. Go for a run, a walk or a bike ride. Find something that suits your personality and fits in your schedule.

Once you choose the simple steps which can lead you to your personal goals, stick to these, and you will see the results almost immediately.

For instance, if you choose to eat healthily, you may opt to prepare your own healthy pack for lunch and snacks at work instead of buying nutritionally vacant foods with too many calories from the vending machine or the workplace cafeteria.

You may prepare for yourself and your family tasty but healthy meals like grilled salmon steak with a meatless sauté of vegetables and a side of boiled organic brown rice. Instead of snacking on pastries or chips laden with sodium and cholesterol, you can choose a snack of grilled Portobello mushroom sandwich, with light cream cheese, lettuce, tomatoes and onion rings and a few soda crackers on the side.

While you are constantly finding ways to keep yourself and your family healthy, try also to keep an open mind. Try to do things you have not tried before deciding it is not for you, like a new sport or a new recipe that cuts the fat and salt by more than half. Keeping yourself healthy and fit is essentially about making the right life choices and keeping them. So always prepare a full plate of healthy yet delicious food and keep going with your personal fitness and healthy lifestyle goals.

As in any new endeavor, it is always best to ease yourself into these new changes. Once you find your groove, keep at it and keep striving to improve yourself. These small changes ultimately add up to vast improvements and lead to a healthier new you in the long run.

Finally, I'd like to thank you for purchasing this book! If you enjoyed it or found it helpful, I'd greatly appreciate it if you'd take a moment to leave a review on Amazon. Thank you!

Printed in Great Britain
by Amazon